Recipe Book/Companion Guide

Foreword/Introduction

This book is meant to complement our feature book entitled "Okinawa Diet: The Ultimate Beginner's Guide for Understanding the Okinawa Diet And What You Need to Know".

That book was written to give you all the information you need before starting the Okinawa Diet, which is known for its tremendously positive effect on life expectancy and vitality. This book contains recipes that follow the guidelines laid out in that book.

There are four major categories for the Okinawa diet: Featherweight, Lightweight, Middleweight, and Heavyweight. These are explained in detail in the Okinawa Beginner's Guide I developed. However, to serve as a refresher of sorts, here is some info:

Featherweight category food items are ideal for those aiming to lose weight, as the ingredients only contain about .08 calories per gram. In this book, we have included Featherweight category recipes featuring food items such as cucumbers, spinach, and tofu, which you can cook to perfection.

In the Lightweight category are recipes that have as much as 1.5 calories per gram. Eat these selected foods for gradual weight loss. These include sweet potatoes and bananas.

Skipping meals is not a recommendation in the Okinawa Diet and neither is starving one's self. The Middleweight category takes care of this aspect for most people. These recipes, despite the relatively higher amount of calories per gram, are still healthy. They complete the traditional Okinawa diet that is appetizing and filling. Lean meat lovers can rejoice in this section. There are also recipes that make use of legumes and high-fiber ingredients.

Recipes that have caloric densities of 9 grams per calorie characterize the Heavyweight category, so avoid consuming these meals frequently if your goal is weight loss.

We wish you exciting days ahead with over 50 recipes to choose from in this recipe book!

Thanks again for grabbing this book. We hope you enjoy it! Dōzo omeshi agari kudasai!

Copyright 2015 by Wade Migan - All rights reserved.

This document is geared towards providing exact and reliable information in regards to the topic and issue covered. The publication is sold with the idea that the publisher is not required to render accounting, officially permitted, or otherwise, qualified services. If advice is necessary, legal or professional, a practiced individual in the profession should be ordered.

In no way is it legal to reproduce, duplicate, or transmit any part of this document in either electronic means or in printed format. Recording of this publication is strictly prohibited and any storage of this document is not allowed unless with written permission from the publisher. All rights reserved.

The information provided herein is stated to be truthful and consistent, in that any liability, in terms of inattention or otherwise, by any usage or abuse of any policies, processes, or directions contained within is the solitary and utter responsibility of the recipient reader. Under no circumstances will any legal responsibility or blame be held against the publisher for any reparation, damages, or monetary loss due to the information herein, either directly or indirectly.

The information herein is offered for informational purposes solely, and is universal as so. The presentation of the information is without contract or any type of guarantee assurance.

The trademarks that are used are without any consent, and the publication of the trademark is without permission or backing by the trademark owner. All trademarks and brands within this book are for clarifying purposes only and are the owned by the owners themselves, not affiliated with this document.

Table of Contents

Chapter 1: Featherweight Recipes

- Spinach Pancakes with Okonomi Sauce

- Soba Noodles with Sweet Potato, Spinach, and Cabbage

- Sweet Potatoes with Spinach and Cashews

- Japanese Yam Pancakes with Bacon and Sesame-Soy Dip

- Tofu Pancakes and Maple Syrup

- Tofu Torinku Soboro (Rice Toppings with Chicken and Bean curd)

- Tofu and Cabbage Gyoza with Soy-Vinegar Dip

- Nihon no Hon with Cabbage

- Baked Tofu in Teriyaki Sauce

- Tofu and Shiitake - Miso Ramen

- Baked Eggplants Glazed in Mirin and Miso

- Prawn and Cucumber Somen Noodles in Iceberg Lettuce Cups

- Hourensou with Ginger Dressing (Spinach Salad)

- Japanese Zucchini with Quinoa and Tomato Soup

- Orange, Cabbage, and Tofu Salad with Balsamic Vinegar Dressing

- Mushroom and Spinach Tofu Omelet

- Grilled Asparagus Tofu Omelet

Chapter 2: Lightweight Recipes

- Sweet Potato Cakes

- Kale and Sweet Potato Smoothie

- Beef and Sweet Potato Japanese Korokke with Tonkatsu Dip

- Shrimps with Sweet Potatoes and Aioli Dip

- Yakitori with Potatoes, Oregano, and Shio Koji

- Fish Tempura and Sweet Potato Wedges

- Glazed Sweet Potato with Soy Sauce and Nori

- Sweet Potatoes Roasts with Scallion Miso Butter

- Tempura-Style Baked Sweet Potatoes

- Choco-Caramel Banana Won Tons

- Sweet Potato Taki Onigiri Wrapped in Nori

- Ingredients

Chapter 3: Middleweight Recipes

- Garlic-Radish Tenderloin Tips with Ponzu Sauce

- Grilled Beef with Cilantro, Tomatoes, and Avocado

- Stir-Fry Beef with Broccoli and Ginger

- Meatballs with Cilantro, Paprika, Cayenne, and Ginger

- Chicken Patties with Hijiki & Edamame

- Stir-Fry Shrimp with Radish and Snow Peas

- Flavorful Adzuki Beans in Tomato-Butternut Squash Soup

- Garlic and Kale with Stir-fry Adzuki Beans

- Spicy Mushrooms, Ginger, and Miso Ramen

- Udon Noodles in Chili Beef-Eye Fillet and Tomatoes

- Soba Noodles with Stir-fried Pork and Sweet Soy Sauce

- 5-Spice Honey Roasted Duck Breast

- Spicy Beef Quinoa with Tomatoes, Black Beans, and Corn Kernels

Chapter 4: Heavyweight Recipes

- Pork Chops with Ginger and Garlic Sauce

- Okinawan Pork Miso with Shoyu Sauce

- Sliced Pork, Bittermelon, and Tofu

- Pan-Grilled Yakiniku Pork Tenderloins

- Braised Pork in Green Onions, Ginger, and Soy Sauce

- Pork Shogayaki with Cabbage Salad and Sesame Dressing

- Cold Soba Noodles with Pork and Garlic Sauce

- Pork Belly in Soy Sauce and Radish

- Gingered Pork Chops in Miso and Sake

- Sesame and Soy Seasoned Pork with Spinach and Carrots

- Stir-Fry Chili Pork Tenderloins

Conclusion

Chapter 1:

Featherweight Recipes

Here are recipes that have a caloric density of around 0.8 calories per gram. Recommended ingredients in the following recipes include cucumbers, spinach, and tofu.

Spinach Pancakes with Okonomi Sauce

Ingredients

    2 cups fresh spinach leaves (chopped)

    3/4 cup water

    1/4 teaspoon salt

    1 cup flour

    Okonomi or Tonkatsu sauce (store-bought)

    1 egg

Directions

In a bowl, add the beaten egg, flour, salt and water, and then mix well until smooth.

In a pan, place the batter and mix the spinach leaves; cover pan to wilt the spinach.

Cook pancakes for 5 minutes on each side; transfer onto a plate.

Serve the pancakes, drizzle Okonomi sauce and enjoy while hot.

Soba Noodles with Sweet Potato, Spinach and Cabbage

Ingredients

    2 small sweet potatoes

    2 tablespoons chives (minced)

    1 bag baby spinach

    6 oz. Soba noodles

    6 cups chicken stock

    2 cups shredded cabbage

    Salt (to taste)

Directions

In a pot, pour the chicken broth, add the cabbage and sweet potatoes, and then simmer for 15 minutes; season with salt.

Add the spinach leaves into the stock, and ladle soup into bowls.

In a small bowl, add the warm Soba noodles; top with the vegetables and garnish with chives.

Sweet Potatoes with Spinach & Cashews

Ingredients

¾ lb. sweet potatoes

2 scallions

1 small ginger

6 oz. baby spinach

2 tablespoons sugar

2 tablespoons sesame oil

¼ cup mirin

1 teaspoon spice blend (recipe below)

¼ cup cashews

⅓ cup sweet white miso paste

Spice Blend Ingredients

- A dash of black sesame seeds
- A dash of white sesame seeds
- ½ sheet of shredded nori
- A dash of ground pepper (freshly ground)

Directions

Preheat your oven to 450 degrees F.

In a medium-sized pot, combine salt, 1 ½ cups water and rice; bring to a boil.

Simmer for 30 minutes until the rice absorbs the liquid, and then set aside.

Meanwhile, in a medium bowl, combine the miso paste, sesame oil, and mirin.

On a sheet pan, place the sweet potatoes and drizzle with olive oil; season it with pepper and salt.

Roast for 24 minutes and transfer to a bowl.

Toss the potatoes with the white bottom scallions and half of the miso mixture.

In a pan, add salt, 2 tablespoons water and salt, and then boil for 3 minutes; add the cashews.

Line another sheet pan with parchment paper, and then transfer the cashews mixture.

In the same sheet pan, cook the ginger with 2 tablespoons of olive oil for 45 seconds; add the spinach leaves, season with pepper and salt.

In a colander, drain excess liquid from the spinach and transfer to the bowl of miso mixture.

On a plate, spread the spinach and sweet potatoes, and top with cashews.

In a small bowl, combine all the spice blend ingredients, garnish on the sweet potatoes and green bottom scallions.

Japanese Yam Pancakes with Bacon and Sesame-Soy Dip

Ingredients

- 3 slices bacon
- 1 1/2 cups yam (finely grated)
- 1 egg
- 1/2 teaspoon salt
- 2 green onions
- 2 tablespoons parsley (finely chopped)

Directions

In a medium-sized bowl, add the grated yam, salt, green onions, parsley and egg.

Whisk to combine the mixture, and set aside.

In a skillet, cook the bacon strips until it turns golden brown; reserve the bacon fat and add the crushed bacon strips to the egg mixture.

In the same skillet, pour a cup of batter and cook until pancake turns brown.

To serve, place the pancakes on a plate and add small dipping bowls of soy sauce and sesame.

Tofu Pancakes and Maple Syrup

Ingredients

    50ml low-fat milk

    100g pancake mix

    1/2 teaspoon cooking oil

    1 egg

    150g soft tofu

    Butter and maple syrup (for garnishing)

Directions

In a bowl, place the strained soft tofu and add an egg; beat until mixture becomes smooth.

Add the pancake mix and low-fat milk, and then mix ingredients.

In a frying pan, add cooking coil and pour portions of the pancake mixture; cook for 5 minutes on each side.

Serve on a plate and add butter or maple syrup on top, if you wish.

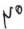

Tofu Toriniku Soboro (Rice Toppings with Chicken and Bean curd)

Ingredients

　　50g chicken

　　2 cups cooked white rice

　　1 teaspoon grated ginger

　　½ tablespoon sake

　　½ tablespoon sugar

　　150g soft tofu

　　½ tablespoon soy sauce

Directions

In a strainer, remove the excess liquid from the soft tofu; transfer into a small bowl.

In separate bowl, mix the soy sauce, sake, sugar, and ginger.

In a pan, stir-fry the chicken with oil and tofu.

Stir in the sake-ginger sauce; toss chicken and tofu to coat.

Place the Soboro on top of a bowl of cooked white rice.

Garnish with parsley and sesame seeds.

Tofu and Cabbage Gyoza with Soy-Vinegar Dip

Ingredients

2 tablespoons sesame oil

1/2 cup quinoa

2 large cloves garlic

1 tablespoon grated ginger

1 tablespoon sake

40 pieces Gyoza wrappers

4 scallions

1/4 teaspoon white pepper

2 dried shiitake mushrooms

1 tablespoon potato starch

1 tablespoons soy sauce

200 grams cabbage

1 pack firm tofu (frozen)

2 tablespoons rice vinegar

1 teaspoon salt

Vegetable oil (for frying)

2 tablespoons soy sauce

Directions

In a pot, boil a cup of water and add the quinoa; remove and add the cabbage.

Use a colander to remove excess water from the cabbage, and transfer to a chopping board to mince.

Combine cabbage with the cooked quinoa and thawed tofu.

In a medium-sized bowl, add the chopped garlic, scallions, soy sauce, sesame oil, salt, potato starch, powdered shitake mushrooms, white pepper and grated ginger.

Fill the Gyoza wrappers with garlic mixture, and seal the edges with water.

Line the dumplings on a parchment paper, and then freeze for 2 hours.

In a frying pan, add 2 tablespoons of vegetable oil; fry the Gyoza until lightly brown.

Serve on a plate, drizzle chili oil on top; combine soy sauce and rice vinegar in a bowl for dipping.

Nihon no Hon with Cabbage

Ingredients

    1 1/2 tablespoon soy sauce (low-sodium)

    1 1/2 lb. frozen scallops

    4 tablespoon breadcrumbs

    3/4 cup mozzarella cheese (low-fat)

    A pinch of sea salt

    1/2 medium cabbage

    1/4 cup parsley

    Olive oil spray

    Ground black pepper

Directions

Preheat your oven to 375 degrees F.

In a skillet, cook the white portion of the cabbage and scallops for about 10 minutes, or until the cabbage turns tender.

Add the green portion of the cabbage and cook for 5 minutes.

Stir in the breadcrumbs, soy sauce, pepper, and salt; cook until sauce thickens.

Coat a small pot dish or casserole with olive oil and add the scallop mixture.

Add the shredded cheese and bake for 10 minutes.

Serve immediately and garnish with parsley.

Baked Tofu in Teriyaki Sauce

Ingredients

1 package tofu (extra firm)

Marinade

4 tablespoons brown rice flour

2 tablespoons tapioca starch

2 tablespoons coconut aminos

2 tablespoons water

1 teaspoon coconut oil

1/2 teaspoon baking powder (gluten-free)

1/2 teaspoon onion powder

1 vegetable bouillon

1/4 teaspoon garlic powder

1/4 teaspoon sesame oil

Sauce

1 tablespoon tapioca starch

1/2 cup pineapple juice

2 tablespoons water

Sesame seeds (for garnish)

1/2 teaspoon sesame oil

1/4 cup coconut aminos

1 chopped spring onion (for garnish)

3 tablespoons maple syrup

1 clove of garlic

Directions

Preheat your oven to 400 degrees F and line a baking sheet with parchment paper.

In a bowl, combine all the marinade ingredients; set aside.

In a colander, place the tofu and press to drain excess liquid.

Place the drained tofu in a bowl, and cut into squares and spread marinade.

Leave the tofu to marinate for 30 minutes at room temperature.

On the baking sheet, line the tofu and bake for 30 minutes.

Meanwhile, in a food processor, add all sauce ingredients and blend until smooth.

In a saucepan, pour the sauce and simmer until thick, and then add the tofu.

Serve the tofu on a plate and garnish with sesame seeds and spring onions.

Tofu and Shiitake-Miso Ramen

Ingredients

- 12 oz. ramen noodles

- 1 pack firm tofu

- 2 scallions

- ¼ cup hoisin sauce

- 6 oz. Choy Sum or Bok Choy

- 2 tablespoons soy sauce

- 2 cloves garlic

- 2 oz. shiitake mushrooms

- 3 tablespoons vegetable stock

- 1 oz. enoki mushrooms

1 tablespoon miso paste

Directions

In a medium-sized pot, add garlic, chopped choy sum and white bottom scallions, and then sauté with vegetable oil for 2 minutes.

Pour in the vegetable stock, 4 cups water, miso, chopped mushrooms, and soy sauce; bring to boil and simmer for 8 minutes.

Meanwhile, in a medium-sized pan, cook the tofu with vegetable oil for 5 minutes.

With the pan still on the burner, but with the heat off, pour the hoisin sauce over the tofu and toss to thoroughly coat. Set aside while you finish the soup.

In the vegetable stock and miso mixture, add the ramen noodles; cook for 4 minutes or until al dente.

In a bowl, ladle the noodles, vegetables and soup; top with tofu.

Garnish with the green scallions, and enjoy while hot!

Baked Eggplants Glazed in Mirin and Miso

Ingredients

    1 ½ lbs. eggplant

    ¼ cup Miso

    1/3 cup scallions

    2 1/2 tablespoons of sugar

    2 tablespoons sake

    2 tablespoons Mirin

Directions

Preheat your oven to 350 degrees F and line foil on a baking sheet.

In a small bowl, mix the miso, sugar, sake and mirin until it forms a thick paste; set aside.

Slice the eggplant into wedges and spread the miso glaze on the baking sheet; cover with another sheet of foil.

Bake for about 25 minutes, remove foil cover and broil eggplants for 10 minutes.

Transfer the caramelized eggplants into a dish and sprinkle with chopped scallions.

Prawn and Cucumber Somen Noodles in Iceberg Lettuce Cups

Ingredients

    1/2 cup coriander leaves

    1 garlic clove (large)

    175g somen noodles
    80ml vegetable oil

    1/2 cup mint leaves

    1 rind and juice of lime

    500g prawns
    2 cucumbers
    Iceberg lettuce

Directions

Boil water in a pot and add the somen noodles; cook until al dente.

Drain the noodles in a colander until it turns dry.

In a bowl, combine the cooked prawns and cucumber slices.

Add garlic, lime rind, lime juice, coriander and mint, and pulse in a food processor.

Gradually pour in the vegetable oil until mixture turns smooth; season it with salt and pepper.

Wash and drain excess liquid from the lettuce; form into cups and add the noodles.

Drizzle some dressing on top and serve.

Hourensou with Ginger Dressing (Spinach Salad)

<u>Ingredients</u>

- 3 tablespoons minced onion
- 3 tablespoons peanut oil
- 2 tablespoons white vinegar
- 1 1/2 tablespoons grated ginger
- 1 tablespoon ketchup
- 1 tablespoon soy sauce (reduced-sodium)
- 1/4 teaspoon minced garlic
- 1/4 teaspoon salt
- Pepper (to taste)
- 10 oz. fresh spinach

1 grated carrot (large)

1 thinly sliced red bell pepper (medium)

Directions

In a food processor, blend the oil, onions, ginger, soy sauce, salt, garlic, pepper, ketchup and vinegar.

In a large bowl, pour the ginger dressing and add the spinach, bell pepper and carrots; toss to evenly coat.

Serve on individual plates and enjoy!

Japanese Zucchini with Quinoa and Tomato Soup

Ingredients

1 tablespoon lemon juice (freshly squeezed)

2 tablespoons olive oil

1 cup zucchini

3 cups water

1 teaspoon coriander (ground)

1 teaspoon oregano (dried)

1 cup diced potato

½ teaspoon pepper

1 ½ cup fresh tomatoes

2 cups onions

½ cup raw quinoa

1 teaspoon salt

1 cup red bell peppers (chopped)

1 teaspoon cumin (ground)

Directions

In a soup pot, heat olive oil and add salt and onions over medium heat.

In a small bowl, rinse the quinoa rice; place a mesh strainer on top to drain.

Once fully drained, transfer the quinoa to the soup pot and combine with oregano, bell pepper, potatoes, cumin, water, coriander and tomatoes.

Cover the soup pot and bring to a boil for around 10 minutes.

Add lemon juice and zucchini in the pot and simmer for 20 minutes until all the vegetables become tender.

Serve the soup while hot and enjoy.

Orange, Cabbage and Tofu Salad with Balsamic Vinegar Dressing

Ingredients

    2 tablespoon balsamic vinegar

    1 1/2 teaspoon olive oil
    1 cup shredded red cabbage
    1 tablespoon pine nuts
    3 oz. firm tofu
    1 cup chopped raw spinach
    1 oz. soft goat cheese
    1/2 cup canned mandarin oranges

Directions

In a large bowl, add the red cabbage, pine nuts, tofu, and the rest of the ingredients.

Gently combine and serve on a plate.

Top with pine nuts and a few pieces of raw spinach.

Mushroom and Spinach Tofu Omelet

Ingredients for the Tofu Omelet

    2 tablespoons nutritional yeast

    2 cloves garlic
    1 package soft tofu

    2 tablespoons olive oil

    1 teaspoon fine black salt (to taste)

    1 tablespoon arrowroot

    1/2 cup chickpea flour
    1/2 teaspoon turmeric

Directions for the Tofu Omelet

    In a food processor, add chopped garlic, nutritional yeast, soft tofu, salt, turmeric, and olive oil; puree until smooth.

Add arrowroot and chickpea flour to the pureed mixture and blend once more.

Preheat a skillet, grease with a bit of oil and pour the omelet batter; cook for 4 minutes before flipping.

Once the omelet reaches the 4th minute, flip it over and cook for a minute longer.

Ingredients for the Filling

Fresh black pepper (to taste)

4 cups sliced white mushrooms

3 tablespoons of fresh thyme (chopped)

2 tablespoons of olive oil

2 garlic cloves

2 cups fresh spinach leaves (chopped)

Salt (to taste)

Directions

In a large pan, sauté the mushrooms and spinach with olive oil for 5 minutes, and then add garlic and thyme.

Sauté the garlic for about 3 minutes more, and then add salt and pepper to taste.

Stuff the spinach and mushrooms in the tofu omelet and top with vegan cheese.

Grilled Asparagus Tofu Omelet

Ingredients for the Tofu Omelet

- 1/2 teaspoon turmeric
- 2 tablespoons nutritional yeast
- 2 cloves garlic
- 1 package soft tofu
- 2 tablespoons olive oil
- 1 teaspoon fine black salt (to taste)
- 1 tablespoon arrowroot
- 1/2 cup chickpea flour

Directions for the Tofu Omelet

In a food processor, add nutritional yeast, turmeric garlic, soft tofu, salt, and olive oil; puree until smooth.

Add chickpea flour and arrowroot with the pureed mixture and blend.

Preheat a skillet, grease with a bit of oil and pour the omelet batter; cook for 4 minutes before flipping.

Flip omelet over and cook for a more minute.

<u>Ingredients for the Filling</u>

- 2 cloves of garlic
- 1 pound asparagus
- ¼ cup balsamic vinegar
- ¼ cup olive oil
- Pepper and salt to taste

Directions for the Filling

In a zip-lock bag, add the asparagus and pour olive oil, vinegar, salt and pepper, and garlic; leave the marinade for 2 hours at room temperature.

Once done, pour the asparagus and marinade in a large pan, and cook for 8 minutes.

Place the filling in the tofu omelet and serve right away with a dash of hot sauce.

Chapter 2:

Lightweight Recipes

Here are recipes that have as much as 1.5 calories per gram. Eat these selected foods for gradual weight loss. Recommended ingredients in the following recipes include spinach, sweet potatoes, and bananas.

Sweet Potato Cakes

Ingredients

    1 teaspoon onion

    1 large egg

    1/8 teaspoon salt

    Ground nutmeg

    1/8 teaspoon pepper

    1 lb. sweet potato

    1/4 cup all-purpose flour

    Cooking spray

Directions

In a small bowl, combine peeled and shredded sweet potatoes, potatoes, all-purpose flour, pepper, salt, egg, and nutmeg.

In a large skillet, grease with cooking spray and add the ingredients.

Toss ingredients to coat the vegetables with the all-purpose flour and cook for about four minutes.

Flatten the cooked sweet potatoes and constantly stir until golden brown.

Serve on a plate and enjoy!

Sweet Potato Bread

Ingredients

    300 grams sweet potato flesh (roasted)

    3 eggs

    1 teaspoon baking soda

    3 tablespoons coconut milk

    Pinch of salt

    1/2 cup coconut flour

    ½ piece of lemon (juiced)

Directions

Preheat oven to 350 degrees F.

Grease a small loaf tin and line with parchment paper.

Set the food processor to pulse mode and fill with all the ingredients.

Spoon the mixture in the tin and smoothen the top with a spoon.

Transfer the tin pan in the oven and bake for 40 minutes.

Open the oven hatch to cover the tin with foil, and then continue baking for 20 minutes.

Once done, remove the tin pan and let it cool before serving in thick slices.

Kale and Sweet Potato Smoothie

Ingredients

1/2 teaspoon of cumin

3 medium sweet potatoes
5 leaves of kale

1 tablespoon coconut oil

½ teaspoon thyme

Directions

Preheat your oven to 375 degrees F.

In a pan, add the cubed sweet potatoes and roast for 45 minutes.

Meanwhile, wash, de-rib and chop the kale leaves into small pieces.

In a separate pan, sauté the kale with coconut oil for 20 minutes.

In the bowl of a food processor, blend the cooled sweet potatoes and kale.

In a tall glass, add 4 ice cubes and pour the potato-kale mixture.

Serve the smoothie and enjoy!

Beef and Sweet Potato Japanese Korokke with Tonkatsu Dip

Ingredients

1 lb. potatoes

1 teaspoon oil

Vegetable oil (for deep-frying)

1/2 minced onion

1 ½ cup bread crumbs

2 eggs

1/2 lb. ground beef

Ground pepper (to taste)

Tonkatsu sauce (store-bought)

¼ teaspoon salt

1 cup flour

Directions

In a pot, add water and boil the sweet potatoes until it's tender.

In a large bowl, mash the potatoes; set aside.

In a pan, sauté the onions, add ground beef; season it with pepper and salt.

Mix the meat and potato mixture and roll into 8 oval-shaped patties; refrigerate for 1 hour.

In a small bowl, place flour and breadcrumbs.

In a separate bowl, add the beaten eggs.

Dip the patties into the egg wash and dredge in the breadcrumb mixture.

Deep-fry the patties for 4 minutes and transfer onto a wire rack or dish lined with paper towels to drain excess oil.

Serve on a plate, add a dipping bowl filled with Tonkatsu sauce and enjoy while hot!

Shrimps with Sweet Potatoes and Aioli Dip

Ingredients

    1 teaspoon ground cumin

    3 baked garlic cloves

    1 large sweet potato

    1/2 roasted yellow bell pepper

    Scallions (for garnishing)

    1/4 cup of corn breadcrumbs

    Pepper and salt (for seasoning)

    3 jumbo shrimps

    Coconut oil (for cooking)

    1/4 cup olive oil

    2 slices red onion

    1/2 roasted red bell pepper

Aioli Sauce Ingredients

    1 lemon

    Salt/Pepper to taste

    4 garlic cloves

    2 red bell peppers

    Extra Virgin Olive Oil (for dressing)

    1 cup mayonnaise

Directions

Preheat your oven to 400 degrees F.

On a baking tray, add the sliced sweet potatoes, and bake for about 40 minutes.

Coat the yellow and red bell peppers with olive oil and spread them on a cookie sheet.

On the same baking tray, add the garlic cloves drizzled with olive oil; bake for 30 minutes.

Remove the garlic and replace it with the shrimps; bake for 10 minutes.

When the shrimps are cooked, season it with pepper and salt.

Meanwhile, place the red pepper on the baking tray and brush it with coconut oil, and then bake for 10 minutes until the skin blackens.

In a food processor, blend the peppers, juice of a lemon, garlic and mayonnaise; season with pepper and salt.

In a bowl of iced water, add the sliced scallions.

In a medium-sized bowl, add the cumin, sweet potatoes, roasted garlic, cumin, pepper, breadcrumbs, bell peppers and salt.

Fold the garlic mixture into the shrimps and roll into small patties; bake for 12 minutes.

Drizzle with the pepper sauce and garnish with scallions and bell peppers.

Serve the shrimp cakes on a plate and add the mayonnaise dip on the side.

Yakitori with Potatoes, Oregano and Shio Koji

Ingredients

- 1 teaspoon paprika

- 1 tablespoon all-purpose flour

- 4 chicken thighs

- 2 cloves garlic

- 1 cup chicken broth

- 1 tablespoon olive oil

- 1/2 teaspoon dried rosemary

- 2 tablespoons Miso Shio Koji marinating seasoning

- 1 small red potato

- 1/2 large onion

- 1 carrot

- 1/4 cup dry white wine

1/2 teaspoon dried oregano

Directions

In a zip-lock bag, insert the chicken, garlic and shio koji; massage the chicken and marinate for 30 minutes.

Soon after, add the herbs, flour and paprika, and then shake the bag to coat the chicken.

In a pan, place the chicken and pour the marinade; cook for 3 minutes per side.

Add onions and sliced carrots; continue cooking for 3 minutes.

Pour the wine, broth and add the potatoes; bring the mixture to a boil.

Simmer for about 40 minutes until chicken and vegetables are tender.

Serve on a plate and enjoy!

Fish Tempura and Sweet Potato Wedges

Tartar Sauce Ingredients

    ½ radish

    175ml. mayonnaise

    3 ½ oz. pickled ginger

    1 teaspoon dried ginger

Tsuyu sauce Ingredients

    2 tablespoons soy sauce

    1 tablespoon mirin

    1 tablespoon pure yuzu (orange) juice

    ½ tablespoon umeboshi (plum) juice

3 tablespoons rice vinegar

4 teaspoons dashi (Japanese stock) concentrates

For the cod

Vegetable oil (for deep-frying)

1 ½ cups flour

2 cups water

2 medium eggs (free-range)

1 lb. cod fillet

For the sweet potato wedges

3 large sweet potatoes

1 tablespoon black sesame seeds

1 tablespoon sea salt

For garnishing

½ small grated radish

Directions

To make the tartar sauce, combine the mayonnaise, radish, and pickled and dried ginger in a small bowl; refrigerate for 1 hour.

To make the Tsuyu Sauce, combine the mirin, yuzu juice, soy sauce, umeboshi juice, rice vinegar and dashi in a small bowl; set aside.

In a baking pan, place the sweet potato wedges and rub salt, and then set aside.

Meanwhile, in a large bowl, mix flour with water and eggs.

In a separate bowl, place the rest of the flour and dredge the cod chunks; dip into the batter.

Fry the cod in batches for three minutes, or until it turns golden brown and crisp.

Drain on paper towels and set aside.

Deep-fry the sweet potato wedges, drain on paper towels and season with ground sea salt and sesame seeds.

Serve the cod and crispy wedges on a plate and garnish with grated radish; in small bowls, pour the dipping sauces alongside.

Glazed Sweet Potato with Soy Sauce and Nori

Ingredients

- 3 tablespoons soy sauce (low sodium)

- 1 sheet shredded nori (toasted)

- 3 sweet potatoes

- 4 garlic cloves

- 1 tablespoon dark sesame oil

- 2 tablespoons brown sugar

- 2 tablespoons mirin

- 1 tablespoon sesame seeds (toasted)

Directions

Preheat your oven to 400 degrees F.

Combine and stir the brown sugar, soy sauce, mirin, garlic cloves, dark sesame oil, and sweet potatoes.

Arrange the potatoes on a baking dish.

Pour soy sauce mixture over the sweet potatoes.

Cover and bake at for about 50 minutes.

Baste the potatoes with the soy sauce mixture; bake for another 10 minutes.

Sprinkle sesame seeds on top together with the nori.

Serve in a bowl and enjoy!

Sweet Potatoes Roasts with Scallion Miso Butter

Ingredients

    8 small slender sweet potatoes

    1 1/2 sticks unsalted butter

    1 1/2 tablespoons miso paste

    3 tablespoons scallions

Directions

Preheat your oven to 450 degrees F.

On a baking sheet, cover with foil and arrange the pricked potatoes; bake for 1 hour.

Meanwhile, in a small bowl, add the miso, butter and scallions.

Serve the sweet potatoes on a plate and garnish with scallion miso butter.

Tempura-Style Baked Sweet Potatoes

Ingredients

    2 teaspoons brown sugar

    3 medium scallions

    1/2 cup and 2 tablespoons olive oil

    1/3 cup soy sauce

    2 medium garlic cloves

    1 tablespoon rice vinegar

    1 cup breadcrumbs

    2 tablespoons mirin

    4 lbs. sweet potatoes

    2 tablespoons fresh grated ginger

Directions

Preheat your oven to 425 degrees F.

In a large bowl, add the soy sauce, mirin, vinegar, garlic, ginger, brown sugar. ½ cup of oil, and cubed sweet potatoes.

In a baking dish, add the potatoes and the mirin mixture; cover with foil and bake for about 20 minutes.

In a pan, add the breadcrumbs and toast it with 2 tablespoons of olive oil. After toasting, remove from pan and set aside.

Remove the baking pan from the oven, remove the foil and roast for 10 minutes until tender.

To serve, sprinkle the sweet potatoes with toasted breadcrumbs and minced scallions.

Choco-Caramel Banana Won Tons

Ingredients

    1 banana

    8 wonton wrappers

    ½ teaspoon sugar

    ¾ cup oil

Garnish Ingredients

    1 tablespoon caramel sauce

    1 tablespoon chocolate syrup

    2 tablespoons chopped nuts

Directions

On a plate, add the chopped bananas and sprinkle sugar on top.

Place one banana in the middle of a wonton wrapper; pink the sides and seal with a dab of water.

In a skillet, add oil and fry the wontons for about 2 minutes until it turns golden brown.

Serve on a plate; drizzle with chocolate sauce, caramel and chopped nuts.

Sweet Potato Taki Onigiri Wrapped in Nori

Ingredients
=

- 1/2 sweet potato

- 3 tablespoons teriyaki sauce (store-bought)

- 1 oz. avocado

- 2 cups water

- 1 tablespoon sesame oil

- 1 tablespoon sesame seeds

- 1 tablespoon honey

- 1 sheet nori

- 1/2 tablespoon freshly ground ginger

- 1 1/2 cups white sushi rice

1/2 teaspoon salt

1 tablespoon sugar

2 tablespoons rice vinegar

Directions

Preheat your oven to 375 degrees F.

In a deep-bottom pan, boil water and add the rice, and then cook for 20 minutes.

In a bowl, mix ginger, sesame oil, honey, and teriyaki sauce; add sliced sweet potatoes.

On a baking sheet, spread the potatoes and coat with the ginger mixture; bake for 20 minutes.

Shape the rice, avocado slices and sweet potatoes into small balls

Dip the rice ball into the ginger mixture; grill on a pan with sesame oil.

Wrap each ball with nori and serve.

Chapter 3:

Middleweight Recipes

Here are recipes that have as much as 3 calories per gram. Consumption of these food items should be done occasionally if gradual weight loss is the goal. Recommended ingredients that are in the following recipes include lean meat, fish, shrimps, legumes, and high-fiber ingredients.

Cold Sesame and Peanut Ramen

Ingredients

- 2 pinches red pepper
- 2 teaspoons ginger
- 1 pound packed ramen noodles
- 2 tablespoons light brown sugar
- 1/4 cup unsalted peanuts
- 4 tablespoons peanut oil
- 4 tablespoons creamy peanut butter
- 2 teaspoons sesame oil
- 1/4 cup green onion tops
- 2 tablespoons soy sauce

Directions

In a medium-sized soup pot, add water and bring to a boil for 8 minutes.

Drain the noodles and transfer it to a large bowl.

In a small mixing bowl, add the ginger, peanut butter, brown sugar, red pepper and sesame oil.

Pour the sesame oil mixture on the pasta and toss it to evenly coat.

Cover the pasta bowl with foil and refrigerate for 2 hours.

Once chilled, serve the ramen and top with chopped nuts and green onions.

Garlic-Radish Tenderloin Tips with Ponzu Sauce

Ingredients

    ¾ lb. tenderloin steak

    Salt (to taste)

    Ground black pepper (to taste)

    2 pieces radish

    1 ½ tablespoons oil

    2 cloves garlic

    2 tablespoons sake

    Scallions (for garnishing)

    3 tablespoon Ponzu sauce (recipe below)

Ponzu Sauce Ingredients

    1 ½ tablespoons miso

    ½ tablespoon rice vinegar

1 tablespoon lemon juice

2 tablespoons soy sauce

1 teaspoon Mirin

Directions

In a bowl, add the grated radish, scallions and garlic.

On a chopping board, trim off excess fat from the tenderloin tips; season it with pepper and salt.

In a frying pan, add oil and sauté the garlic until lightly brown.

Transfer the garlic on paper towels to drain excess oil; retain garlic oil in the pan.

Cook the steak in the pan until it turns brown, and then flip to continue cooking the other side.

Pour sake and shake pan to distribute evenly.

Place the tenderloin tips on a plate, and then garnish with grated radish, crunchy garlic and scallions.

In a small bowl, combine all the ingredients for the sauce; pour over the grated radish garnish, crunchy garlic flakes and scallions.

Serve immediately and enjoy!

Grilled Beef with Cilantro, Tomatoes and Avocado

Ingredients

    6 cups torn mixed salad greens

    1 small avocado

    1/2 cup Shio Koji seasoning

    2 tablespoons fresh cilantro

    1/4 teaspoon ground black pepper

    1/2 teaspoon lime peel

    1/4 cup onion (chopped)

    2 small yellow tomatoes

    12 oz. beef flank steak

Directions

Preheat your oven to 160 degrees F.

In a zip-lock bag, insert the steak and place it on a shallow dish; set aside.

In a screw-lid jar, add the lime peel, Shio Koji and cilantro; cover and shake.

In the jar, add the onions, cover and shake then add with the steak; marinate overnight.

The following day, remove the bag from the refrigerator and discard the marinade.

Transfer the steak on a broiler pan; sprinkle with pepper.

Broil the steak in the oven for 18 minutes, or depending on your preferred doneness.

Once done, remove the steak from the oven and transfer on a chopping board to slice it across the grain.

On a plate, arrange the avocado slices and tomatoes; top with the steak.

Drizzle the remaining Shio Koji and serve.

Stir-Fry Beef with Broccoli and Ginger

Ingredients

    8 oz. beef top round steak

    1/2 cup beef broth (reduced-sodium)

    3 tablespoons soy sauce (reduced-sodium)

    2 1/2 teaspoons cornstarch

    1 teaspoon sugar

    1/2 teaspoon fresh ginger

    Cooking spray

    12 oz. fresh or frozen asparagus

    1 1/2 cups sliced fresh mushrooms

    1 cup small broccoli florets

    4 green onions

    2 teaspoons olive oil

2 cups cooked brown rice

Directions

Start this recipe by trimming off excess fat from the round steak.

Prepare the sauce by getting a small bowl to mix the cornstarch, soy sauce, sugar, ginger and beef broth.

Set the first few ingredients aside and cook the vegetables.

Coat a large skillet with cooking oil and add the mushrooms, green onions, broccoli florets and asparagus.

Cook for about 5 minutes to soften the vegetables, and then, once done, serve on a plate.

In the same skillet, add the meat and olive oil; stir-fry the sliced round steak for 3 minutes, add the sauce and cook until done.

Get the plate you set aside and add all the vegetables in the skillet.

Cook for 2 minutes to heat the sauce, and serve with cooked rice.

Meatballs with Cilantro, Paprika, Cayenne and Ginger

Meatball Ingredients

    1 egg

    1 pound ground beef
    1 small finely chopped onion

    1/4 teaspoon ground ginger

    2 tablespoons fresh cilantro (minced)

    1 tablespoon paprika

    3 tablespoons fresh parsley (minced)

    2 tablespoons ground cumin
    1/4 teaspoon cayenne pepper
    1/2 teaspoon cinnamon
    1/2 teaspoon pepper

Ingredients for the Sauce

1 cup of beef broth (organic)

2 tablespoons olive oil
2 cups crushed organic tomatoes

2 medium chopped onions

1/2 teaspoon black pepper

1/2 cup parsley (freshly chopped)

4 minced garlic cloves
2 teaspoons ground cumin

1/2 cup parsley (freshly chopped)
Pinch of cayenne

Directions

In a large bowl, mix all meatball ingredients and roll them into large balls.

Drizzle coconut oil and place the balls in a skillet pan; cook for 15 minutes until golden brown.

Prepare a pot to cook the sauce and set heat to medium-high.

Add olive oil, garlic, pepper, onions, parsley, cayenne and cumin.

Cook for about 10 minutes, then add the cooked meatballs and simmer for 15 minutes.

Serve the spicy meatballs in a bowl and enjoy!

Chicken Patties with Hijiki & Edamame

Ingredients

    2 teaspoons dried Hijiki seaweeds

    A handful of Edamame

    300g ground chicken

    1 egg

    2 teaspoons soy sauce

    1 tablespoon potato starch

Flavoring Ingredients

    2 tablespoons soy sauce

    2 tablespoons Mirin

2 tablespoons cooking sake

1 tablespoon sugar

Directions

Before starting, re-hydrate the Hijiki and thaw the Edamame.

In a bowl, add the minced chicken, hijiki, egg, edamame, soy sauce and

Add the hijiki and edamame from Step 1, and the minced chicken, egg, soy sauce and potato starch to a bowl.

In a pan, add vegetable oil and add the bite-sized chicken and hijiki.

Pour in the flavoring ingredients; simmer and reduce the sauce.

Coat the chicken patties or tsukune with the reduced sauce.

Serve on a plate and enjoy!

Stir-Fry Shrimp with Radish and Snow Peas

Ingredients

    20g radish

    100ml water

    30g snow peas

    2/3 teaspoon olive oil

    2 tablespoons shrimp

    1 tablespoon sake

    2 pinches of salt

    ½ teaspoon pepper

Directions

In a medium-sized bowl, soak the radish in water for about 5 minutes; transfer radish to a pan but reserve liquid.

In a pan, stir-fry the shrimp; add the snow peas, salt, water, sake, and pepper.

Pour the reserve radish liquid into the pan and simmer.

Serve the shrimps and vegetables on a plate and enjoy!

Flavorful Adzuki Beans in Tomato-Butternut Squash Soup

<u>Ingredients</u>

- 4 cups diced butternut squash

- 5 whole tomatoes (canned)

- 1 teaspoon coriander

- 1 teaspoon cinnamon

- ½ teaspoon grated ginger

- 6 garlic cloves

- 1 piece dried Japanese kelp

- 2 medium onions

- 4 cups dried adzuki beans

- 5 ½ cups water

2 teaspoons salt

~~2 teaspoons chipotle pepper~~

1 tablespoon chopped parsley

2 tablespoons olive oil

Directions

In a large pot, add olive oil to sauté the squash, onions, garlic, cinnamon, salt and coriander; add 5 cups water and boil for 10 minutes.

Mash the squash and add the tomatoes; simmer before adding the adzuki beans.

Cook until the beans turn soft; serve in a bowl and garnish with cilantro.

Garlic and Kale with Stir-fry Adzuki Beans

Ingredients

6 cups kale leaves

1 teaspoon ground cumin

1 tablespoon olive oil

1/4 cup tamari — Soy

1 cup adzuki beans (uncooked)

Salt (to taste)

1 teaspoon ground coriander

2 cloves garlic

2 tablespoons water

Pepper (to taste)

Directions

In a medium-sized saucepan, add the beans and boil with about 3 cups of water, and simmer for 45 minutes.

In a medium-sized skillet, add water and sauté garlic and kale; season with cumin, coriander and tamari.

Stir the beans, reduce the heat and continue to simmer for another 20 minutes.

Serve the beans and kale soup in a bowl; season with pepper and salt.

Spicy Mushrooms, Ginger and Miso Ramen

Ingredients

200g ramen noodles

3 spring onions

1 red chili

½ carrot

250ml chicken stock

1 tablespoon miso paste

Small thumb ginger

100g mushrooms

250ml water

1 teaspoon rice vinegar

½ stick lemongrass

Directions

In a pot, simmer the miso paste, chicken stock and water.

Add the carrots, spring onions, chili, ginger, mushrooms and lemongrass, and cook for about 10 minutes.

Drop the ramen noodles in the same pot and cook until al dente.

Strain the cooked noodles and transfer to a plate; allow it to dry.

Transfer the noodles to a wide-mouthed bowl and add hot soup and rice vinegar.

Garnish with parsley and enjoy!

Udon Noodles in Chili Beef-Eye Fillet and Tomatoes

Ingredients

    1 clove garlic

    2 tablespoons Balsamic vinegar

    100g Sun-dried tomatoes (in oil)
    60g butter

    750g Beef-eye fillet
    ½ teaspoon chili paste

    360g Udon noodles
    2 tablespoons Balsamic vinegar

    Olive oil
    2 tablespoons basil leaves

Directions

In a jar with a lid, add the chopped sun-dried tomatoes, vinegar and oil, shake well and set the vinaigrette aside.

In a large bowl, add the chopped beef and marinate with the vinaigrette.

In a pan, grill the beef with oil until it turns golden brown.

Remove beef from heat and allow it to rest for 10 minutes; slice beef into thin strips.

Boil water in a pot and cook the Udon noodles until al dente.

In a bowl, combine the garlic, chili paste, half of the tomatoes and butter.

In a colander, drain the Udon and run through cold water.

Once noodles turn dry, pour in the chili-butter and garlic mixture and serve on a bowl.

Top the beef slices over the Udon and drizzle the remaining vinaigrette.

Soba Noodles with Stir-fried Pork and Sweet Soy Sauce

Ingredients

    1 medium onion

    1 tablespoon sesame oil 70g Soba noodles
    300g Pork
    2 tablespoon olive oil
    60ml of Mirin

    500g Bok choy
    1 clove garlic
    2 tablespoons sake

    1 red bell pepper 60ml soy sauce

    1 tablespoon Sugar
    1/2 sheet Nori

    1 teaspoon grated ginger

Directions

In a pot of boiling water, add the Soba noodles, and then cook until al dente.

Transfer noodles in a colander, run through cold water, drain and set aside.

In a wok, add pork and stir-fry with sesame oil, and cook until brown.

Transfer meat into a bowl, cover to keep warm.

In a saucepan, add the soy sauce, sake, sugar and miri.

Stir well until sugar dissolves.

In the same wok, pour the remaining oil and sauté garlic, ginger, and onions.

Add the bok choy and chopped red bell pepper.

Mix in the noodles, pork, pickled ginger and sweet soy sauce.

Toss to coat and serve on a plate.

5-Spice Honey Roasted Duck Breast

Ingredients

    2 teaspoons honey

    2 lbs. boneless duck breast

    2 oranges (Zest & juice)

    1 teaspoon five-spice powder

    1/4 teaspoon cornstarch

    1 tablespoon soy sauce (reduced-sodium)

Directions

Preheat your oven to 375 degrees F.

Place the duck on a cutting board with its skin side facing down.

Trim off excess skin, make diagonal cuts, and then sprinkle five-spice powder.

In a skillet, place the duck and cook until golden brown; transfer to oven.

Roast the duck for 15 minutes. Once done, transfer to a cutting board to rest for 5 minutes.

In the same skillet, pour the duck fat from the pan and simmer with honey and orange juice.

Add in the soy sauce and orange zest and cook until sauce reduces.

Add in the cornstarch and stir until mixture is thick.

Transfer the duck to a plate, thinly slice it and serve with the orange sauce.

<u>Ingredients for the Five-Spice Seasoning</u>

    1 1/2teaspoons fennel seeds

6 pieces of star anise

3/4 teaspoon ground garlic cloves

3 tablespoons cinnamon

1 1/2 teaspoons whole black peppercorns

Directions for the Five-Spice Seasoning

Combine all the ingredients in the blender until they are finely ground.

Spicy Beef Quinoa with Tomatoes, Black Beans and Corn Kernels

Ingredients

- 2 cups water

- 1 can crushed tomatoes

- 1 teaspoon dried parsley

- 1 lb. lean ground beef

- 1 jalapeno pepper

- 1 onion

- 1 green bell pepper

- 1 cup frozen corn kernels

- 1 tablespoon olive oil

- 1 tablespoon ground cumin

1 cup uncooked quinoa

4 cloves garlic

1 tablespoon chili powder

1 red bell pepper

1 zucchini

2 cans black beans

1 teaspoon dried oregano leaves

Ground black pepper

Salt

1/4 cup chopped fresh cilantro

Directions

In a saucepan, add water and bring it to a boil.

Mix in the quinoa and simmer it for about 20 minutes until it fully absorbs the water.

In a large skillet, cook the ground beef until it turns brown, and then remove excess fat and set aside.

Prepare a large pot and add olive oil to cook the garlic, onions and jalapeno peppers for about 5 minutes.

After 5 minutes, add cumin and chili powder to the pot and drop the black beans, tomatoes, zucchini, parsley, oregano and bell peppers.

While cooking the vegetables for 20 minutes, lower the heat and simmer the quinoa and corn kernels.

Once the vegetables have softened, turn off the oven and use a ladle to serve the Spicy Beef Quinoa with Tomatoes, Black Beans and Corn Kernels.

Garnish with extra cilantro leaves.

Chapter 4:

Heavyweight Recipes

Here are recipes that have as much as 9 calories per gram. The recommended ingredients in the following recipes include oils, nuts, and red meat.

Pork Chops with Ginger and Garlic Sauce

Ingredients

    A handful of fresh cilantro

    2 tablespoons vegetable oil

    4 small pork chops

Dressing Ingredients

    1 ½ tablespoons granulated sugar

    ¼ cup light soy sauce

    2 tablespoons ginger

    2 tablespoons garlic

    1 teaspoon sesame oil

    1 jalapeno

    2 tablespoons safflower oil

¼ cup rice wine vinegar

Directions

In a small bowl, combine all the dressing ingredients; set aside.

In a large pan, add the safflower oil and fry the pork chops for about 3 minutes per side.

Transfer the chops on a plate and pour the soy mixture.

Serve with a garnish of cilantro and cooked rice.

Okinawan Pork Miso with Shoyu Sauce

Ingredients

    2 teaspoons crushed garlic

    2 1/4 lbs. of pork butt
    2 teaspoons crushed ginger
    1/2 cup Shoyu sauce (soy sauce)

    3/4 cup water

    Cilantro leaves (for garnishing)
    3 tablespoons of miso
    1/4 cup sugar

    A shot of sake

Directions

Preheat your oven to 350 degrees F.

In a zip-lock bag, place the pork butt and sake; marinate for 1 hour.

Transfer the pork in a pot, boil water and add the ginger; cook for 2 hours.

In a small saucepan, add the Shoyu, sugar, pork butt and sake, and then bake for 45 minutes.

Once the pork butt turns tender, serve it on a plate and garnish with cilantro.

Sliced Pork, Bittermelon, and Tofu

Ingredients

    1/2 lb. sliced pork

    1/2 lb. firm tofu

    1 egg

    2 bitter melon

    1/2 medium onion

Spices

    1 teaspoon smoked, dried fish

    1/2 teaspoon salt

    1 tablespoon sake

    1/2 teaspoon sesame oil

    1 1/2 tablespoons soy sauce

Directions

Preheat your griller.

On a chopping board, slice the bitter melons or goya, and then remove the seeds.

Sprinkle salt and massage the entire fruit; set aside for 5 minutes.

In cooking paper, wrap the sliced tofu; microwave for about 2 minutes.

Grill the tofu for another 2 minutes; transfer on a plate.

In a pan, sauté the Goya and onions for about 3 minutes, and then add the pork.

Pour soy sauce, sake and the smoked, dried fish.

Mix the egg and grilled tofu and serve on a plate.

Pan-Grilled Yakiniku Pork Tenderloins

Ingredients
===

- 1 1/2 tablespoons soy sauce

- 2 garlic cloves

- 1/2 lb. pork tenderloin (about 230 grams)

- 1/4 teaspoon dry mustard

- 1 1/2 tablespoons sesame oil

- 1 tablespoon rice vinegar

- 1 1/2 tablespoons sugar

- Pepper (to taste)

- 1 1/2 tablespoons mirin

- 1 1/2 tablespoons roasted sesame seeds

1 1/2 tablespoons miso

Directions

In a pan, add the sesame seeds, roast them, and remove after the third popping sound.

In a mortar and pestle, grind the roasted seeds and transfer to a bowl.

Add in the soy sauce, dry mustard, rice vinegar, sugar, pepper, mirin, miso and minced garlic.

Marinate the pork tenderloins with the soy mixture, and refrigerate for 8 hours.

Grill the pork slices and serve on a plate.

Braised Pork in Green Onions, Ginger and Soy Sauce

Ingredients

    ½ ginger

    3 tablespoons green onions (chopped)

    ¾ lb. pork belly

    ½ tablespoon oil

    1 teaspoon salt

Seasonings

    1/3 cup soy sauce

    1/3 cup sake

    2/3 cup water

3 tablespoons sugar

Directions

In two small bowls separate the green and white bottoms of the green onions.

Soak the white bottom green onions in cold water for about 10 minutes; drain all liquid.

Place the pork belly slices on a plate and rub with salt.

In a skillet, add oil and cook the fat-side for about 10 minutes until it turns brown.

Meanwhile, in a pot, add water, sake, sugar and soy sauce.

Place the pork belly, ginger, green onions and ginger; bring to a rolling boil.

Cook the pork belly for about 1 hour; leave at least ¼ liquid to prevent pork belly from burning.

Remove meat from the pot, transfer to a plate, and then cut into slices.

Serve the meat with ramen noodles or rice.

Pork Shogayaki with Cabbage Salad and Sesame Dressing

Ingredients

- 3 tablespoons mirin

- 1 tablespoon oil

- 7 oz. pork loin chunks

- 2 tablespoons sake

- 1 head of cabbage (shredded)

- 2 tablespoons soy sauce

- 2 tablespoons ginger root

Sesame Dressing

5 tablespoons mayonnaise

1 tablespoon rice vinegar

2 teaspoons soy sauce

2 teaspoons sugar

1/2 teaspoon salt

2 tablespoons ground sesame seeds

2 teaspoons sesame oil

Directions

In a bowl, mix grated ginger, sake, soy sauce and mirin, and then set aside.

In a frying pan, add sliced pork and fry with oil; add the ginger mixture to coat.

In a bowl, mix all the cabbage salad's dressing until it turns smooth.

Serve the pan-fried meat on a plate and add shredded cabbage on the side.

Liberally drizzle the sesame dressing on the salad and enjoy!

Cold Soba Noodles with Pork and Garlic Sauce

Ingredients

    2 tablespoon rice wine

    2 stalks spring onions

    270g Soba noodles
    1 tablespoon mirin

    1 teaspoon chili oil

    2 small pork fillets (raw)
    ½ cup coriander sprigs

    1 tablespoon fresh ginger
    2 tablespoon extra-virgin olive oil

    1 teaspoon sugar
    2 cloves garlic
    2 tablespoon dark soy

Directions

In a pan, combine spring onions, rice wine, ginger, olive oil and pork slices.

In a small bowl, mix the sugar, soy, mirin, chili oil and garlic.

Toss the garlic mixture with the Soba noodles.

In a single-serve deep bowl, add the pork slices, Soba noodles and pour more sauce if you wish.

Garnish with coriander sprigs and enjoy!

Pork Belly in Soy Sauce and Radish

Ingredients

- 20 pieces dried sardines
- 600g pork belly
- 1 teaspoon salt
- 2 large cloves
- 1 tablespoon granulated sugar
- 1 1/2 cups water
- 1 tablespoon soy sauce
- 1/3 cup sake
- 45g ginger

Instructions

In a pot, add the pork belly, and fry in its own fat until it turns golden brown.

Transfer to a plate and set aside.

In a pan, add the garlic, ginger, and dried sardines; fry in pork belly fat until golden brown.

Pour in the sake in the sardine mixture.

In a bowl, mix the sugar, salt, soy sauce and water; pour into the pot and simmer.

Return to the pot and simmer the pork belly for 2 hours until meat is tender.

In a colander, strain the braising liquid and remove excess fat.

Serve on a plate, pour the braising liquid on the pork, and then garnish with hot mustard and steamed vegetables of choice.

Gingered Pork Chops in Miso and Sake

Ingredients

    2 tablespoons granulated sugar

    330g pork chops

    3 tablespoons miso

    1 tablespoon grated ginger

    4 tablespoons sake

    Sesame dressing (store-bought)

Directions

In a large bowl, combine the sugar, miso, ginger and sake.

Dip each pork chop slice in the miso-ginger marinade, and then transfer to a tray.

Pour the remaining marinade on the tray; set aside.

In a frying pan, place the marinated pork slice and fry until golden brown.

Serve on a plate and add shredded cabbage, drizzle with sesame dressing.

Sesame and Soy Seasoned Pork with Spinach and Carrots

Ingredients

    1 tablespoon sesame seeds

    ¼ slice of carrot

    A bunch of spinach leaves

    1 tablespoon sesame oil

    100g ground pork

Seasoning Ingredients

    1 tablespoon soy sauce

    1 tablespoon sake

    1 tablespoon sugar

Directions

On a chopping board, slice the carrot into very thin strips, and then transfer into a bowl and microwave for 1 minute.

In a pot, boil the spinach leaves with water; shock in a bowl of iced water.

In a colander, drain the spinach leaves and julienne.

In a pan, add sake, sugar, soy sauce and ground pork, and stir-fry until brown.

In a bowl, add the spinach and carrot strips, pour soy sauce mixture and meat.

Serve on a plate and pair with a bowl of rice.

Stir-Fry Chili Pork Tenderloins

Ingredients

- 8 scallions

- 1 red bell pepper

- 2 tomatoes

- 1 jalapeño pepper

- 2 garlic cloves

- 2 teaspoons fresh ginger

- 4 teaspoons soy sauce

- 1 teaspoon sesame oil

- 2 teaspoons canola oil

- 1 pound pork tenderloin

- 1 can of pineapple chunks

¼ cup fresh cilantro (chopped)

2 cups white rice (cooked)

Directions

In a skillet, add the canola oil, stir-fry the pork tenderloin for about 2 minutes, and then transfer to a plate.

In the same skillet, add the first 8 ingredients; stir-fry until tender.

Toss the pork with the vegetables, garnish with cilantro and serve with white rice.

Conclusion

Thank you again for grabbing both of our books on the Okinawa diet. This diet has helped so many people over the years. There is no doubt in my mind that these recipes can assist you in reaching whatever your health and fitness goals are, from weight loss to muscle gain.

If you've enjoyed any of these recipes in particular, please take the time to share your thoughts by sending me a personal message, or even posting a review on Amazon. It would be greatly appreciated and I try my best to get back to every message!

The next step is to mix and match these recipes within the given categories of the Okinawa diet program. Good luck, or gambatte ne!

Made in the USA
San Bernardino, CA
04 May 2019